BYE ACNE!

All About Acne and Simple Way to Overcome It

Kingster

Kingster

Acknowledgement

I'd like to thank my understanding, supportive parents and wife for their help which allowed me to fully focus on the book write-up. It's tough to juggle between work, family, a demanding toddler and study. But you've made things better and easier for me to cope during this period.

CONTENTS

CHAPTER 1
What is Acne

Acne is a common skin condition that affects nearly 10% of the world's population and up to 50 million American yearly. At least 85 percent of people in the U.S. experience acne between the ages of 12 and 24 years. However, acne is not only limited to teenagers who undergoing hormonal changes but also it affects other ages.

Acne is a disorder that affects the skin's oil glands and hair follicles. While sometimes it seems pimples appear overnight, the development of an acne breakout is an extended process that begins at the cellular level. All pimples begin as a blockage of the hair follicle, or pore. Gaining an understanding of why a blockage begins and how a pimple develops will ultimately help you in treating your acne.

The small holes in skin (pores) connect to oil glands under the skin. These glands make an oily substance called sebum. The pores connect to the glands by a canal called a follicle. Inside the follicles, oil carries dead skin cells to the surface of the skin. A thin hair also grows through the follicle and out to the skin. Sometimes, the hair, sebum, and skin cells clump together into a plug that obstructs the pore opening. This obstruction is called a comedo. It manifests itself as non-inflamed bump or blackhead on the skin's surface. The bacteria in the plug cause swelling. Then when the plug starts to break down, a pimple grows. Acne is usually not a serious health threat, but it can cause scars. Acne lesions include whiteheads, blackheads, small bumps, and nodules and cysts.

The early stage of acne starts with whiteheads (clogged pores not open to the surface and medically known as closed comedones) and blackheads (clogged pores open to the surface and medically known as open comedones) which are non-inflammatory acne.

When whiteheads rupture the hair follicle wall, pimples are formed when solidified sebum, dead cells from the pore and bacteria are released into the skin. This is the stage called inflammatory acne. If pimples become infected, the infection may penetrate deep into the skin and form cysts (cystic acne) which are painful lumps. The cysts may rupture and leave temporary or permanent scars and post-inflammatory pigmentation (dark spots). Cysts may become as large as 2,5 cm across. A patient with acne may show only non-inflammatory lesions or a combination of non-inflammatory and inflammatory lesions with or without scars and brown spots.

Below is the summary of types of acne:

a)   Whiteheads: These remain under the skin and are small
b)   Blackheads: Clearly visible, they are black and appear on the surface of the skin
c)   Papules: Small, usually pink bumps, these are visible on the surface of the skin
d)   Pustules: Clearly visible on the surface of the skin. They are red at their base and have pus at the top
e)   Nobules: Clearly visible on the surface of the skin. They are large, solid, painful pimples that are embedded deep in the skin

f)   Cysts: Clearly visible on the surface of the skin. They are painful and filled with pus. Cysts can cause scars.

CHAPTER 2
Who and When is affected by Acne

I t's easy to associate acne with youth. Hormonal changes, pubescence, teenage oily skin, stress, and poor diet in our early 20s—these are all things commonly linked to acne. Acne can occur at any age. If underlying factors are not addressed, acne may not stop at all. Twenty-six percent of 40-year-olds and 12% of 50-year-olds suffer from acne, and 10% of females have oily skin from puberty on through their whole life.

Acne is an extremely common skin condition in adolescence. It occurs in both sexes, although teenage boys tend to have the most severe cases. Women are more likely than men to have mild to moderate forms into their 30s and beyond. Girls typically start to get acne when their hormones kick in (approximately 11 to 13 years old), which is about the time that they start their period. Boys start to get acne at the age of approximately 12 years, with a range of 9 to 15 years old. As most girls will attest, boys on average mature later than girls. The age that adolescents start to get acne is different in each adolescent and the severity may differ from person to person. Asking the adolescent's biological parents when they started having acne may be a good way to predict when she/he will get acne and may give a clue to how serious the acne will be. Acne in babies is uncommon and results from the effect of maternal hormones. Most people outgrow acne; but in women it may last until the menopause. 5% of women of 40 years of age have acne; but only 1% of men in that age group.

The main lesions of teen acne are blackheads and whiteheads. Later in puberty, there is a higher incidence of inflammatory lesions. Blackheads and whiteheads (non-inflammatory acne) may develop into pimples or pustules (inflammatory acne), and pimples may develop into cysts. Teenagers are usually active and have very busy school and after-school schedules as well as increasingly active social lives. Being a teenager is tough enough as it is without adding the complicating factor of acne. Unfortunately, one pimple can make the difference between popularity and outcast in the mind of many teens.

CHAPTER 3
Where is acne

A cne is a condition of the skin and it can show up on any part of the body. Some areas of the body are more prone to develop acne including on your face, neck, chest, shoulders, back and upper arms. These areas have a higher percentage of sebaceous glands, which produce sebum. When bacteria mix with sebum near these glands, an acne lesion can form. Areas of thicker skin, like the palms of the hands and soles of the feet do not develop acne; however, it is possible for acne to appear on the genital regions. While these areas are less common, some people have more sebaceous glands than others and may be prone to acne on any portion of the skin with a high percentage of these glands. The severity may differ from person to person and may fluctuate over time. Acne often has an adverse emotional effect on sufferers.

The face was the main location where most young people had acne. This is due to there a lot of sebaceous glands there. Young people thought this was a difficult place because it's often visible. Some people found their acne affected all parts of their face, for others there were specific bits. This included:

a) T zone (forehead and/or nose)
b) Cheeks
c) Jawline

d) Chin

e) Ears/earlobes

f) Hairline and scalp.

The parts of face affected by acne could change on a day-by-day basis.

Some people had acne on their back and shoulders as well as their face. This had extra difficulties, like:

a) reaching to apply topical creams

b) pain whilst lying down

c) blood on clothes and bedding from popped spots

d) pain when clothes pressed on back spots (tight tops, bra straps)

e) embarrassment wearing some clothes (like summer/ beach clothes, backless dresses)

f) others seeing the back acne (e.g. when changing for PE classes at school)

Since your skin can tell you so much about your health, it's always a good idea to pay attention to what the location of your acne means, as well as what type of acne it is, in order to get a better idea of what's going on inside your body. If it seems like new or worsening acne is cropping up — despite taking care of your health and your hygiene — it may be one way to tell if something greater is going on with your health.

While most acne is simply due to clogged pores, it's possible that it might be a sign of something else. It is important to consider your skin's natural tendencies as new acne develops. If acne is common for you, that's one thing, but if your acne suddenly becomes worse, consider any other changes in your health or medications and get help from your medical professional or see a dermatologist.

Acne could be a sign of a hormonal imbalance, a side effect of medications you're taking, or even a symptom of a yeast infection, or other systemic issues. Depending on where the acne is, it can be easier to pin down the cause. Here are few places acne can crop up and what it may mean, according to experts.

1. Lower Face/Chin/Neck

If acne is appeared your lower face, neck, and chin before the start of your period, or after emotional stress, experts say there's a good chance your hormones are imbalanced. This type of acne may be more cystic with deep, painful, red nodules. Since it's so deep, cystic acne can take a long time to heal, and often leaves behind red or brown scars. By the time they seem to fade, another cycle of hormonal lesions may be on the rise, leading to a sense that acne is present throughout the month. Picking or squeezing cystic acne is so tempting but it can increase the chance of scarring. Instead, you might want to ask your doctor for oral contraceptives, which can help moderate your hormones and prevent this type of acne.

2. Forehead

The body can react to unhealthy levels of stress by breaking out in blemishes anywhere on the body, but most commonly on the forehead. The connection between stress and acne is the rise in cortisol levels which leads to overactive sebum, creating clogged pores and acne. Sebum is what clogs your pores as it combines with substances such as bacteria and dead skin cells on the surface of the skin resulting in breakouts. Stress acne is typically associated with the forehead, however, it can pop-up anywhere depending on the cortisol levels and the other environmental factors associated with the stress. But no need to worry if stress is causing acne to crop up for you — speaking with your dermatologist can help you find solutions on how to manage it.

3. Around the Mouth

Hormonal acne around your mouth and lips can be a sign of other issues. It often is not a tell for a serious underlying disorder, but if seen with other symptoms, your doctor may want to work up for polycystic ovarian syndrome (PCOS). Other symptoms of PCOS include thinning hair on your scalp, irregular periods, depression, and fertility issues. If you have acne around your mouth, it doesn't mean you have PCOS, but if it's accompanied by these other symptoms, it may be worth looking into as a possible cause.

4. Face/Back/Buttocks

If you notice new acne popping up on your face, chest, back, or buttocks, it could be a side effect of your prescription medication. These medications include testosterone, progesterone, steroids, lithium, phenytoin, isoniazid, vitamins B2, B6, and B12, halogens, and epidermal growth factor inhibitors. Management of acne that is caused by drugs includes standard acne therapy. Discontinuation of the offending drug may be necessary in some cases.

5. Chest

Chest acne is another one that's common among teenagers. But if you're past those hormonal years, and still have chest pimples, a different skin condition may be to blame. Acne most commonly affects the face, back, and chest, so chest acne is not necessarily different than face acne. However, there is another condition called folliculitis, which is basically inflammation of the hair follicles and has a number of different causes, that can occur on the chest and looks very similar to acne. Your dermatologist can determine what it is and offer the correct form of treatment.

6. Bikini Line

If you have bumps that look like pimples around your vaginal area, it could also be due to folliculitis. Folliculitis can be caused by a variety of factors such as tight clothing, friction, sweat, hair removal, excess oil, harsh or irritating skin care products, and infectious organisms. Even ingrown hairs can cause folliculitis, but in that case, there is usually a hair in the bump. Allergic or irritant reactions can also cause acne-like bumps.

While acne in these places doesn't guarantee you have another health issue going on, it's always a good idea to monitor your body for changes, and to speak with a doctor if something feels off.

CHAPTER 4
Why is Acne

Hormonal factors

Acne is primarily a hormonal condition driven by male or 'androgenic' hormones, which typically become active during the teenage years. Sensitivity to such hormones, combined with bacteria on the skin, and fatty acids within oil glands, cause acne. Common sites for acne are the face, chest, shoulders, and back -- the sites of oil glands.

Increased production of oil stimulated by androgenic (male sex) hormones. During the teens, hormones stimulate hair growth, as well as oil secretion by the sebaceous glands. Hormonal changes can stimulate sebaceous glands to produce more sebum. Therefore, anything that raises hormone levels (for example pregnancy, stress, menstrual periods and certain medicines, such as corticosteroids) could aggravate acne. The male sex hormone testosterone, which is present in both men and women, is mainly responsible, but the female sex hormone progesterone also contributes to acne in women.

(Some babies are born with acne because their mothers pass certain hormones on to them just before birth. This is rare and usually self-limiting.)

Oily (Greasy) Skin

People with acne often have an oily (greasy) skin. It starts when greasy secretions from the skin's sebaceous glands (oil glands) plug the tiny openings for hair follicles (plugged pores). If the openings are large, the clogs take the form of blackheads: small, flat spots with dark centers. If the openings stay small, the clogs take the form of whiteheads: small, flesh-colored bumps. Both types of plugged pores can develop into swollen, tender inflammations or pimples or deeper lumps or nodules.

Obstruction of the opening of the follicle caused by increased production of scales (keratin)

Infection by a bacterium, namely Propionibacterium acnes. The bacteria Propionibacterium acnes and Staphylococcus epidermis occur naturally in hair follicles. If there are too many bacteria, they may secrete enzymes that break down sebum, promoting inflammation in the follicle. Some people may be more sensitive to this reaction than others, making their acne more severe.

Foods

Some foods that can cause acne and why the quality of your diet is important as below:

1. Refined Grains and Sugars

People with acne tend to consume more refined carbohydrates than people with little or no acne.

Foods rich in refined carbohydrates include:

Bread, crackers, cereal or desserts made with white flour

Pasta made with white flour

White rice and rice noodles

Sodas and other sugar-sweetened beverages

Sweeteners like cane sugar, maple syrup, honey or agave

One study found that people who frequently consumed added sugars had a 30% greater risk of developing acne, while those who regularly ate pastries and cakes had a 20% greater risk. This increased risk may be explained by the effects refined carbohydrates have on blood sugar and insulin levels. Refined carbohydrates are absorbed quickly into the bloodstream, which rapidly raises blood sugar levels. When blood sugars rise, insulin levels also rise to help shuttle the blood sugars out of the bloodstream and into your cells.

However, high levels of insulin are not good for those with acne. Insulin makes androgen hormones more active and increases insulin-like growth factor 1 (IGF-1). This contributes to acne development by making skin cells grow more quickly and by boosting sebum production.

On the other hand, low-glycemic diets, which do not dramatically raise blood sugars or insulin levels, are associated with reduced acne severity. While the research on this topic is promising, more is needed to further understand how refined carbohydrates contribute to acne.

2. Dairy Products

Many studies have found a link between milk products and acne severity in teenagers.

Two studies also found that young adults who regularly consumed milk or ice cream were four times more likely to suffer from acne.

However, the studies conducted so far have not been high-quality. The research to date has focused mainly on teenagers and young adults and has only shown a correlation between milk and acne, not a cause and effect relationship.

It is not yet clear how milk may contribute to the formation of acne, but there are several proposed theories. Milk is known to increase insulin levels, independent of its effects on blood sugar, which may worsen acne severity. Cow's milk also contains amino acids that stimulate the liver to produce more IGF-1, which has been linked to the development of acne.

Although there is speculation on why drinking milk may worsen acne, it is unclear whether dairy plays a direct role. More research is needed to determine if there is a specific amount or type of dairy that may aggravate acne.

3. Fast Food

Acne is strongly associated with eating a Western-style diet rich in calories, fat and refined carbohydrates. Fast food items, such as burgers, nuggets, hot dogs, french fries, sodas and milkshakes, are mainstays of a typical Western diet and may increase acne risk.

One study of over 5,000 Chinese teenagers and young adults found that high-fat diets were associated with a 43% increased risk of developing acne. Regularly eating fast food increased the risk by 17%. A separate study of 2,300 Turkish men found that frequently eating burgers or sausages was linked to a 24% increased risk of developing acne.

It is unclear why eating fast food may increase the risk of developing acne, but some researchers propose that it may affect gene expression and alter hormone levels in a way that promotes acne development.

However, it is important to note that most of the research on fast food and acne has used self-reported data. This type of research only shows patterns of dietary habits and acne risk and does not prove that fast food causes acne. Thus, more research is needed.

4. Foods Rich in Omega-6 Fats

Diets containing large amounts of omega-6 fatty acids, like the typical Western diet, have been linked to increased levels of inflammation and acne. This may be because Western diets contain large amounts of corn and soy oils, which are rich in omega-6 fats, and few foods that contain omega-3 fats, like fish and walnuts.

This imbalance of omega-6 and omega-3 fatty acids pushes the body into an inflammatory state, which may worsen acne severity.

Conversely, supplementing with omega-3 fatty acids may reduce levels of inflammation and has been found to reduce acne severity. While the links between omega-6 fatty acids and acne are promising have been no randomized controlled studies on this topic, and more research is needed.

Research suggests that the severity and frequency of acne depend on the strain of bacteria. Not all acne bacteria trigger pimples. One strain helps to keep the skin pimple-free.

Hygiene

Greasy or oily substances may develop acne where your skin comes into contact with oily lotions and creams or with grease in a work area, such as a kitchen with fry vats.

Acne isn't caused by dirty skin. In fact, scrubbing the skin too hard or cleansing with harsh soaps or chemicals irritates the skin and can make acne worse.

Cosmetics

Cosmetics don't necessarily worsen acne, especially if you use oil-free makeup that doesn't clog pores (non-comedogenics) and remove makeup regularly. Non-oily cosmetics don't interfere with the effectiveness of acne drugs.

Other Factors

People of all ages can get acne, but it's most common in teenagers.

Family history. Genetics plays a role in acne. If both parents had acne, you're likely to develop it, too.

Friction or pressure on your skin. This can be caused by items such as telephones, cellphones, helmets, tight collars and backpacks.

Stress doesn't cause acne, but if you have acne already, it may make it worse. Stress may aggravate acne but cannot cause it. Acne may cause stress.

CHAPTER 5
How to Treat Acne

N o treatment is needed for the occasional pimple or two, but if acne causes you distress, something should be done about it. Many different treatments are available, but not each is appropriate for everyone. It is therefore important to keep appointments with your health care provider so that, together, you can determine the right treatment for you. Treatment usually shows an effect only after six to eight weeks.

There is no cure for acne, but effective treatment is available. Severe acne requires medical treatment.

Acne may be mild (few, occasional pimples), moderate (inflammatory papules), or severe (nodules and cysts). Treatment depends on the severity of the condition.

Acne may cause embarrassment, frustration and anger, and sufferers tend to withdraw from school and social activities. Acne certainly impairs quality of life.

Diagnosis
Acne is easily diagnosed by physical examination and medical history.

When signs of androgen excess are present such as menstrual irregularity, hair loss on the scalp and hair growth on the body, specialist referral is essential to exclude overproduction of androgenic hormones by the ovaries or adrenal glands.

The diagnosis of acne is usually straightforward, but acne-like lesions may be caused by systemic medication (eg. cortisone), cortisone applied to the face, and, greasy cosmetics.

Rosacea is characterised by redness, red bumps and pimples. Comedones are absent. Patients are usually middle aged.

Medication

There are many over-the-counter medications (creams, lotions, and gels) available. Many of them contain benzoyl peroxide, alpha-hydroxy acids or salicylic acid. These medications should be water-based and hypoallergenic.

For non-inflammatory acne the treatment of choice is tretinoin (Retin A, retinoic acid), a vitamin A derivative, or adapalene (Differin) or benzoyl peroxide 5% (Panoxyl) in the evening. Both Retin A and Panoxyl may cause redness, burning and scaling (= irritation effect), and sensitivity to sunlight. When this occurs, apply the medication every second evening until the skin settles.

For mild inflammatory acne a topical antibiotic (such as Eryderm) may be added for application in the morning.

For moderate inflammatory acne a systemic (oral) antibiotic, such as tetracycline, is the treatment of choice. Minocycline is preferred by most dermatologists (dosage 50 mg to 100 mg per day). Alternative systemic antibiotics include erythromycin, clindamycin and sulphonamides. Topical treatment (tretinoin included) should be continued to combat inflammation. Be aware, though, that antibiotics may make women susceptible to yeast infections.

Oral antibiotics may be prescribed for up to 6 months for patients with moderate to severe acne. These aim to lower the population of P. Acnes. The dosage will start high and reduce as the acne clears. P. acnes can become resistant to the antibiotic in time, and another antibiotic is needed. Acne is more likely to become resistant to topical rather than oral antibiotics. Antibiotics can combat the growth of bacteria and reduce inflammation. Erythromycin and tetracycline are commonly prescribed for acne.

The tetracycline group of drugs causes yellowing of the teeth if taken after the third month of pregnancy. These drugs should be stopped if you become pregnant and only started again following the completion of breast-feeding. Tetracyclines must not be given to children before the permanent teeth have erupted because these drugs can cause yellow discolouring of permanent teeth.

For marked inflammatory acne (deep, chronically inflamed cysts), the drug isotretinoin (Roaccutane) may be prescribed. This drug has potentially severe side-effects during pregnancy and the treatment must be monitored.

The rate of cure is between 70 and 80% after five months of treatment. All forms of treatment should be continued for a minimum of three months.

If the condition shows improvement the current therapy regimen may be continued. If not, modification of treatment should be considered.

An anti-androgenic contraceptive pill (Diane-35) may be useful in some women with inflammatory acne.

Triamcinolone, a type of corticosteroid, may be injected directly into cysts. This drug may darken the skin around the lesion.

Surgery

Dermatologists can surgically remove scars associated with acne. Three techniques are available: dermabrasion, chemical peeling, and laser resurfacing. These treatments are used to remove scarred skin, exposing the underlying, unblemished skin layers.

Foods

Foods and nutrients that may help keep your skin clear:

Omega-3 fatty acids: Omega-3s are anti-inflammatory, and regular consumption has been linked to a reduced risk of developing acne.

Probiotics: Probiotics promote a healthy gut and balanced microbiome, which is linked to reduced inflammation and a lower risk of acne development.

Green tea: Green tea contains polyphenols that are associated with reduced inflammation and lowered sebum production. Green tea extracts have been found to reduce acne severity when applied to the skin.

Turmeric: Turmeric contains the anti-inflammatory polyphenol curcumin, which can help regulate blood sugar, improve insulin sensitivity and inhibit the growth of acne-causing bacteria, which may reduce acne.

Vitamins A, D, E and zinc: These nutrients play crucial roles in skin and immune health and may help prevent acne.

Paleolithic-style diets: Paleo diets are rich in lean meats, fruits, vegetables and nuts and low in grains, dairy and legumes. They have been associated with lower blood sugar and insulin levels.

Mediterranean-style diets: A Mediterranean diet is rich in fruits, vegetables, whole grain, legumes, fish and olive oil and low in dairy and saturated fats. It has also been linked to reduced acne severity.

It is probably not necessary to completely avoid all the foods that have been linked to acne but rather consume them in balance with the other nutrient-dense foods discussed above. The research on diet and acne is not strong enough to make specific dietary recommendations at this time, but future research is promising.

In the meantime, it may be beneficial to keep a food log to look for patterns between the foods you are eating and the health of your skin. You can also work with a registered dietitian for more personalized advice.

Topical treatments

Tea-tree oil: Results of a study of 60 patients published in the Indian Journal of Dermatology, Venereology, and Leprology suggested that 5-percent tea-tree oil may help treat mild to moderate acne. Gels containing at least 5 percent tea tree oil may be as effective as lotions containing 5 percent benzoyl peroxide, although tea tree oil might work more slowly. Possible side effects include minor itching, burning, redness and dryness. Tea tree oil should be used only topically.

Bovine cartilage. Creams containing 5 percent bovine cartilage, applied to the affected skin twice a day, may be effective in reducing acne.

Tea: There is some evidence that polyphenols from tea, including green tea, applied in a topical preparation, may be beneficial in reducing sebum production and treating acne. However, the compounds in this case were extracted from tea, rather than using tea directly.

Moisturizers

Moisturizers: These can soothe the skin, especially in people who are using acne treatment such as isotretinoin, say researchers. Moisturizers containing aloe vera at a concentration of at least 10 percent or witch hazel can have a soothing and possibly anti-inflammatory effect. Creams and lotions are best for sensitive skin. Alcohol-based gels dry the skin and are better for oily skin.

Corticosteroid injection

If an acne cyst becomes severely inflamed, it may rupture. This can lead to scarring.

A specialist may treat an inflamed cyst by injecting a diluted corticosteroid. This can help prevent scarring, reduce inflammation, and speed up healing. The cyst will break down within a few days.

Self-Care

Apple cider vinegar is made by fermenting apple cider, or the unfiltered juice from pressed apples. Like other vinegars, it is known for its ability to fight many types of bacteria and viruses. Apple cider vinegar contains several organic acids that have been shown to kill P. acnes. Succinic acid has been shown to suppress inflammation caused by P. acnes, which may prevent scarring. Also, lactic acid has been shown to improve the appearance of acne scars. What's more, apple cider vinegar may help dry up the excess oil that causes acne in the first place. It is important to note that applying apple cider vinegar to your skin can cause burns and irritation, so it should always be used in small amounts and diluted with water.

Zinc is an essential nutrient that's important for cell growth, hormone production, metabolism and immune function. It is also one of the most studied natural treatments for acne. Research shows that people with acne tend to have lower levels of zinc in their blood than those with clear skin. Several studies have shown that taking zinc orally helps reduce acne. In one study, 48 acne patients were given oral zinc supplements three times per day. After eight weeks, 38 patients experienced an 80–100% reduction in acne. The optimal dosage of zinc for acne has not been established, but several studies have shown a significant reduction of acne using 30–45 mg of elemental zinc per day. Taking too much zinc may cause adverse effects, including stomach pain and gut irritation. It is also important to note that applying zinc to the skin has not been shown to be effective. This may be because zinc is not effectively absorbed through the skin.

Make a Honey and Cinnamon Mask where both honey and cinnamon are excellent sources of antioxidants. Studies have found applying antioxidants to the skin is more effective at reducing acne than benzoyl peroxide and retinoids. These are two common acne medications for the skin that have antibacterial properties. The antioxidants studied were vitamin B3, linoleic (omega-6) fatty acid and sodium ascorbyl phosphate (SAP), which is a vitamin C derivative. These specific antioxidants are not found in honey or cinnamon, but there is a possibility that other antioxidants may have a similar effect. Honey and cinnamon also have the ability to fight bacteria and reduce inflammation, which are two factors that trigger acne. While the anti-inflammatory, antioxidant and antibacterial properties of honey and cinnamon may benefit acne-prone skin, no studies exist on their ability to treat acne.

Moisturize with Aloe Vera whose leaves produce a clear gel. The gel is often added to lotions, creams, ointments and soaps. It's commonly used to treat abrasions, rashes, burns and other skin conditions. When applied to the skin, aloe vera gel can help heal wounds, treat burns and fight inflammation. Aloe vera also contains salicylic acid and sulfur, which are both used extensively in the treatment of acne. Several studies have shown that applying salicylic acid to the skin significantly reduces acne.

Exfoliation is the process of removing the top layer of dead skin cells. It can be achieved mechanically by using a brush or scrub to physically remove the cells. Alternatively, it can be removed chemically by applying an acid that dissolves them. Exfoliation is believed to improve acne by removing the skin cells that clog up pores. It is also believed to make acne treatments for the skin more effective by allowing them to penetrate deeper, once the topmost layer of skin is removed. Unfortunately, the research on exfoliation and its ability to treat acne is limited. Some studies show that microdermabrasion, which is a method of exfoliation, can improve the skin's appearance, including some cases of acne scarring. In one small study, 25 patients with acne received eight microdermabrasion treatments at weekly intervals. Based on before and after photos, this helped improve acne. 96% of the participants were pleased with the results and would recommend the procedure to others. Yet while these results indicate that exfoliation may improve acne, more research is needed. There are a wide variety of exfoliation products available in stores and online, but it's just as easy to make a scrub at home using sugar or salt.

The hormones released during periods of stress may increase sebum production and skin inflammation, making acne worse. In fact, multiple studies have linked stress to an increase in acne severity. What's more, stress can slow wound healing by up to 40%, which may slow the repair of acne lesions. Certain relaxation and stress-reduction treatments have been shown to improve acne, but more research needs to be done. Get more sleep, engage in physical activity, practice yoga, meditate and take deep breaths to reduce stress.

Exercise promotes healthy blood circulation. The increase in blood flow helps nourish the skin cells, which may help prevent and heal acne. Exercise also plays a role in hormone regulation. Several studies have shown that exercise can decrease stress and anxiety, both of which are factors that can contribute to the development of acne. It's recommended that healthy adults exercise for 30 minutes 3–5 times per week. This can include walking, hiking, running and lifting weights.

For acne-prone skin during breakouts, it's important to protect against sun exposure. Ultraviolet rays stimulate pigment producing cells, increasing the risk of acne scarring. The best option is to use natural sunscreens and to only get an appropriate amount of direct sun exposure daily (about 15–20 minutes most days). Commercial sunscreens are packed with harmful chemicals that can irritate sensitive skin and acne-prone skin. Research shows that coconut oil has an SPF value of 8, as does olive oil. To use as sun protection, apply a moderate amount to exposed skin every couple of hours and try to avoid spending too much time in direct sunlight during "peak" hours, which is about from 10am-3pm each day.

Manuka honey comes from New Zealand where the manuka bush is indigenous. So-called "active" manuka honey is widely promoted on the Internet as an acne remedy. The claim is mostly based on studies that suggest it has significant antibacterial and wound-healing properties. In one study, researchers observed that honey-impregnated wound dressings have gained increasing acceptance in hospitals and clinics worldwide. But they also pointed out it's unclear how they work. So they investigated the ability of three different types of honey to quench the production of free radicals. In their report, they stated that manuka honey was the most effective. On the Internet, patient testimonials about manuka honey's effects on acne range from glowing to dismissive. To date, however, there have been no definitive studies to prove or disprove the effectiveness of manuka honey.

Tannins or fruit acids have natural astringent properties. They can be gotten by boiling a mixture of 5 to 10 grams of extract of bark from such trees as witch hazel, white oak, or English walnut in one cup of water. Commercial preparations, though, are not recommended. The distillation process removes the tannins. Fruit acids include citric, gluconic, gluconolactone, glycolic,malic, and tartaric acids. These have natural properties that help them remove skin.

Jojoba oil is a natural, waxy substance extracted from the seeds of the jojoba shrub. The waxy substances in jojoba oil may help to repair damaged skin, which means it may also help speed up wound healing, including acne lesions. Some of the compounds in jojoba oil might help to reduce skin inflammation, which means it may reduce redness and swelling around pimples, whiteheads, and other inflamed lesions. In a 2012 study, researchers gave 133 people clay face masks that contained jojoba oil. After 6 weeks of using the masks 2 to 3 times per week, people reported a 54 percent improvement in their acne.

Many traditional medicine practitioners use garlic to treat infections and boost the body's ability to fight germs and infections. Garlic contains organosulfur compounds, which have natural antibacterial and anti-inflammatory effects. Organosulfur compounds can also help to boost the immune system, which helps the body fight infections. To fight the inflammation and infections caused by acne, people can add more garlic to their diet. Some people chew whole garlic cloves, rub it on toast, or make it into a hot drink. People can also buy garlic powders or capsules from most grocery stores and natural health stores. Although many online sources recommend that people apply garlic directly to pimples, this may cause further skin irritation. Garlic can burn the skin, so always use it carefully.

Green tea is high in antioxidants that can help to reduce inflammation in the skin. Green tea contains high concentrations of a group of polyphenol antioxidants called catechins. Most people with acne have too much sebum, or natural body oils, in their pores and not enough antioxidants. Antioxidants help the body break down chemicals and waste products that can damage healthy cells. Green tea may help clear out some of the debris and waste that has built up in open acne sores. Green tea also contains compounds that may help to reduce the skin's sebum production, reduce P. acnes and reduce inflammation. Green tea might help either when people drink it or use green tea extract on their skin, though researchers say that the current evidence is limited. However, one study found a 79 and 89 percent reduction in whiteheads and blackheads after 8 weeks of using polyphenol green tea extract. People can find green tea in most high street stores. Green tea extract is harder to find, but it is available from some health stores or online.

Echinacea, Echinacea purpurea, also known as the purple coneflower, may contain compounds that help destroy viruses and bacteria, including P. acnes. Many people believe that Echinacea can boost the immune system and reduce inflammation and use it to fight off or prevent infections, including colds and flus. People can apply creams containing Echinacea to areas where they have acne lesions or take Echinacea supplements. Echinacea products are available from health stores or online as creams or supplements.

Rosemary extract, or Rosmarinus officinalis, contains chemicals and compounds that have antioxidant, antibacterial, and anti-inflammatory properties. Few studies have looked at the effect of rosemary extract on acne, but a 2013 study on mice models and human cells suggested that rosemary extract can reduce inflammation from the acne-causing bacteria P. acnes.

Purified bee venom has been shown to contain antibacterial properties. In a 2013 study, researchers found that purified bee venom can destroy P. acnes bacteria. People who used cosmetics with purified bee venom for 2 weeks had improvements in the number of acne lesions. In a 2016 study, people who applied a gel containing purified bee venom to their face for 6 weeks saw a reduction in mild to moderate acne lesions. Purified bee venom may be a useful future ingredient in acne medication, though more research is needed.

Like other natural remedies, coconut oil contains anti-inflammatory and antibacterial compounds. These properties mean that coconut oil may destroy acne-causing bacteria and reduce redness and swelling of pimples. Coconut oil may also speed up healing in open acne sores. Try rubbing pure, virgin coconut oil directly to the area with acne. Look for coconut oil in the natural foods section of grocery stores or online.

Along with home remedies, specific lifestyle changes can have a powerful effect on keeping the body healthy, making the skin less oily, and reducing acne flare-ups. Lifestyle changes to improve acne include:

- Never touching pimples

People should avoid touching acne sores as doing so can cause further infections. It can be very tempting, but touching acne sores will irritate the skin, may make the pimple worse, and can spread pimples to other areas. Touching, rubbing, squeezing, or popping acne sores can also introduce more bacteria into the lesion, causing further infections. Squeezing a pimple can push bacteria and debris further into the skin, so the pimple may come back worse than it was before. Talk with a doctor about large sores or those that are deep under the skin to find out how to remove them safely.

- Choosing the right cleanser

Many regular soaps have an acidity, or pH, that is too high and can irritate the skin, making acne worse. Choose cleansers, rinses, and washes with a pH closer to the skin's natural pH of around 5.5 to reduce the risk of acne flare-ups and let sores heal.

- Using oil-free skincare

Oil-based or greasy products can block pores, increasing the risk of them becoming clogged and forming acne sores. Look for skin care products and cosmetics labeled as 'oil-free' or 'non-comedogenic,' which contain ingredients that allow pores to breathe.

- Staying hydrated

Staying hydrated is extremely important because it makes it easier for acne sores to heal and reduces the overall risk of outbreaks. When the skin is dry, it can easily become irritated or damaged, resulting in pimples. Being hydrated also ensures new skin cells develop correctly as sores heal. There is no standard daily recommend water intake because each person's water needs are different, depending on age, how active they are, temperature, and any medical conditions. Many health authorities recommend drinking between six and eight 8-ounce glasses of fluid daily.